GW00792310

First published 2009

Published by
Professor Grace Dorey
Old Hill Farm, Portmore, Barnstaple, Devon, EX32 0HR, UK
Telephone: +44 (0) 1271 321721
Email: grace.dorey@virgin.net
www.yourpelvicfloor.co.uk

ISBN 978-0-9545393-5-1

Pump Up Your Penis

This little book is for men of all ages. And that means you! Whether you call it the droop, erectile dysfunction, or simply "can't get it up", the inability to get an erection probably isn't something you talk about a lot. But many men will experience erection problems at some point, so it's worth finding out what you can do right now so that you may both cure and prevent it. Just a few simple daily exercises can keep your pelvic floor healthy, firm up your erection and prevent future problems. A big crane needs a strong base, so read on and pump those muscles!

Grace Dorey

Contents

Section 1: Getting to know your tackle

The long and short of erection problems

Let it all hang out

Erection, know thyself

Meet your muscles

Whatever turns you on

Reaching the finish line

What goes up must come down

Losing you libido

When willies don't work

Do your tackle a favour

All in the mind?

It really does happen to lots of men

Section 2: Working your sex muscles

How flexing your muscles can help

Use it or lose it!

How to give your pelvic floor a workout

Do I have to lie down?

How many exercises should I perform?

Pump before exertion

How long till my fella gets up?

Section 3: Visiting a sex clinic

It's good to talk
Going to a clinic
Testosterone patches
Sex pill for men
Injections
Vacuum therapy
Sexual pain
Pump it up!

Section 1: Getting to know your tackle

The long and short of erection problems

Sometimes, things don't work the way we want them to. Many men find they can't get an erection at some point in their lives, or it's not as firm as they'd like it to be. In this book we're going to take an informative and light-hearted look at your pelvic floor, and find out how to keep your tackle in good working order.

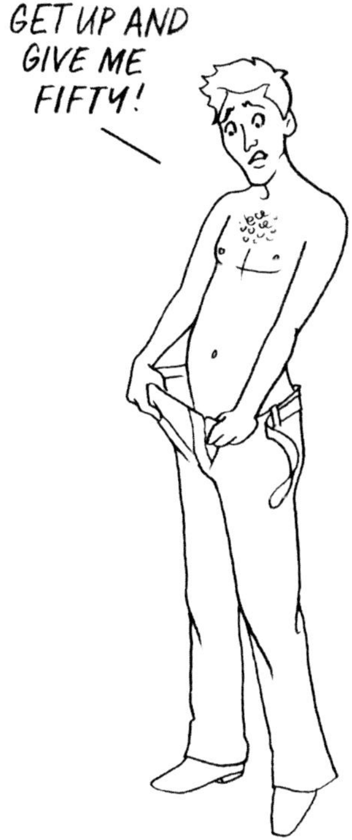
GET UP AND
GIVE ME
FIFTY!

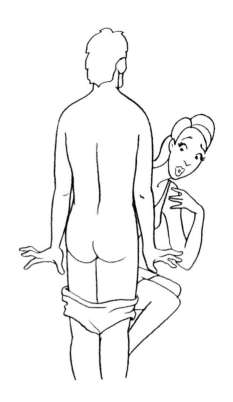

Let it all hang out

I bet you probably realised this already, but most men have one penis and two testicles. One diligent student even gained a PhD viewing the testicles on Greek sculptures; he found that sometimes the left testicle hung lower (51%), and sometimes the opposite was true (22%), or they were of equal height (27%). You don't have to go off and examine any sculptures (unless you really want to) but it might be helpful to start off with a look at your own equipment.

Erection, know thyself

Let's start with the bits you can see. Did you know that your penis has two cavities within it? They're not the kind of cavities you need to see a dentist about though! These cavities fill up with blood when you get turned on and cause an erection.
If you keep your pelvic floor pumped and healthy, the muscles prevent blood from escaping from the cavities and help you keep your erection firm until after orgasm.

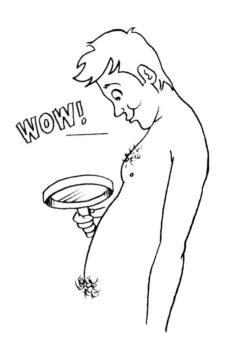

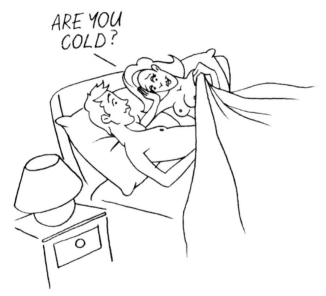

Meet your muscles

Now for the bits you can't see. Your pelvic floor is a group of muscles that has the important job of keeping your insides where they belong and controlling your bladder and bowels. You also have a cremaster muscle which is responsible for raising your testicles when they are touched, aroused, or enter cold water.

Whatever turns you on

All sorts of things can turn you on and trigger an erection. These include sight, smell, sound, touch, taste, erotic thoughts and memories, or a combination of different things. Triggers are different for each man depending on their experiences, sexual preference, relationship and age.

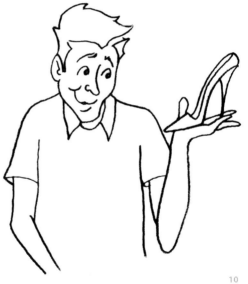

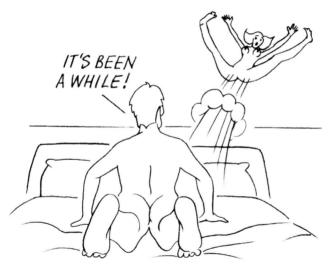

Reaching the finish line

When sexual stimulation gets really intense, the muscles in your pelvic floor pump rhythmically. It's part of the reaction that causes ejaculation. Strong pelvic floor muscles can lead to increased orgasm, so it's worth keeping them fit and toned.

What goes up must come down

Sometimes you come before you want to, which can be frustrating for you and your partner. If this happens regularly, try identifying the point of no return so you can step down the stimulation. Some men find they can delay their orgasm by relaxing their pelvic floor muscles. That's another good reason for understanding how your muscles work.

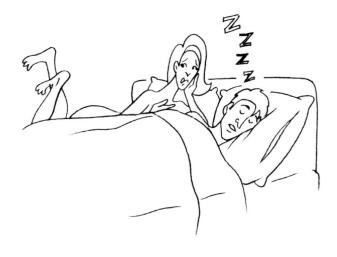

Losing your libido

You need a good helping of testosterone to make you feel sexy. As men age, their body produces less testosterone. If you lose your desire and you have a hormone deficiency, it can be sorted out by wearing a patch containing testosterone gel. You'll need to make sure the patch doesn't come into contact with your partner, particularly if she is, or might be, pregnant.

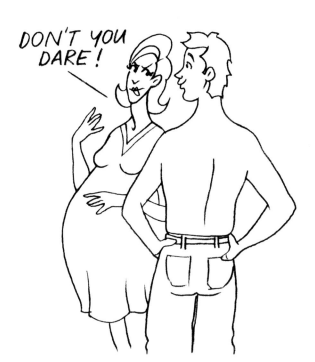

When willies don't work

 You might have heard it called "brewer's droop", but too much booze isn't the only thing that can stop you getting it up. Insufficient blood flow, nerve damage, hormone imbalance, trauma from surgery or radiotherapy, side effects from medication, smoking, drug abuse and weak pelvic floor muscles can all cause problems.

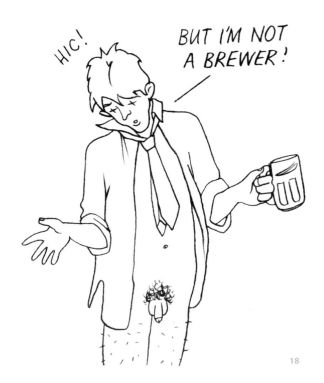

Do your tackle a favour

Sometimes your tackle is trying to tell you something. Not being able to get an erection can be a sign of things like diabetes and heart disease. So it's worth doing yourself and your willy a favour and booking an appointment with your GP.

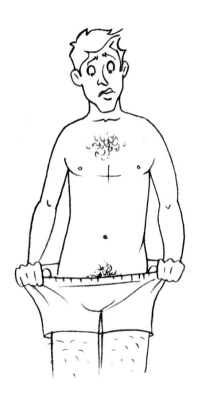

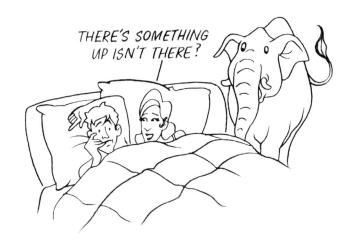

All in the mind?

Your mind plays a really important part in getting an erection. Things like stress, worries, phobias, gender identity issues and an over-strict upbringing can all prevent you from getting an erection. If you're worried, it's worth seeing your GP or talking to a Counsellor who has experience of working with people with sexual problems.

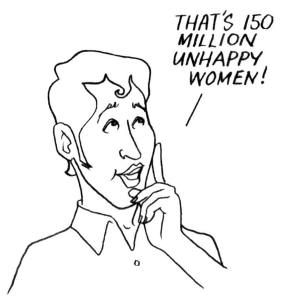

It really does happen to lots of men

Many men experience problems getting an erection. We don't
have any exact figures, probably because no-one likes to talk
about it! But the people who study this sort of thing estimate
that erectile dysfunction affects 150 million men worldwide.
That's more than twice the population of Great Britain,
so you're definitely not alone.

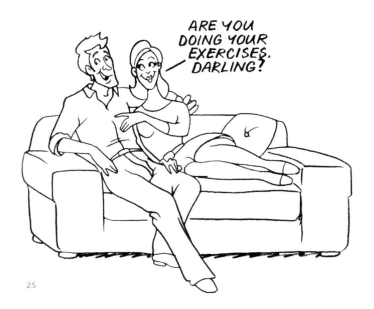

How flexing your muscles can help

Research conducted in 2004 showed that 40% of men with erection difficulties regained normal erections after performing regular pelvic floor exercises. A further 35% saw improved function. That's got to be worth flexing for!

Use it or lose it!

Like any muscles, your pelvic floor muscles will weaken if you don't use them. Regular exercises can get them in good shape again. A Specialist Physiotherapist can perform a gentle examination to assess how strong your pelvic floor is.

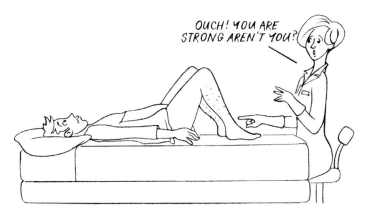

How to give your pelvic floor a workout

Tightening your pelvic floor muscles is easy. Just lie on your back with your knees bent and slightly apart. Now squeeze your muscles as if you were trying to stop a pee and trying to stop wind escaping. You should feel the base of your penis move towards your body, and your testicles rise a bit. Hold the contraction as strongly as you can without tensing your buttocks or holding your breath.

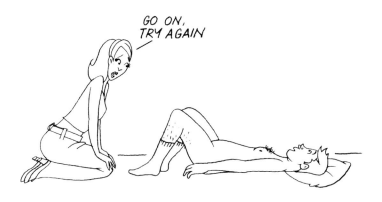

Do I have to lie down?

You can flex your pelvic floor in any position you like. Of course, some positions are easier than others, and it's best to find one that works for you. Many men find it easiest to work their pelvic floor muscles while sitting or standing, with knees and feet apart.

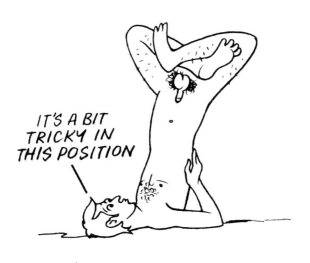

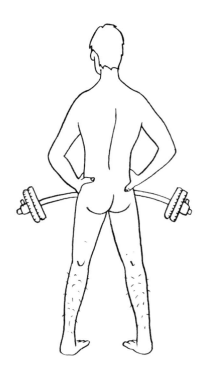

How many exercises should I perform?

Twice a day perform 3 contractions in each position – standing, sitting, and lying down. Hold each contraction for up to 10 seconds, followed by a 10 second rest. That's only 18 contractions a day to firm up your erection and get your tackle fit and healthy!

Pump before exertion

It's a good idea to tighten your pelvic floor muscles before any activity that increases pressure in your abdomen. That includes coughing, sneezing, lifting, shouting, bending and getting out of a chair. You can also lift your pelvic floor up slightly when walking.

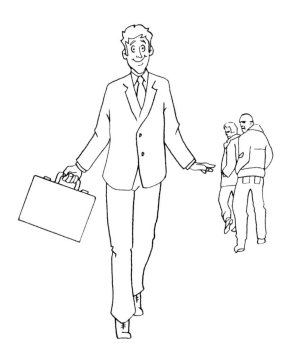

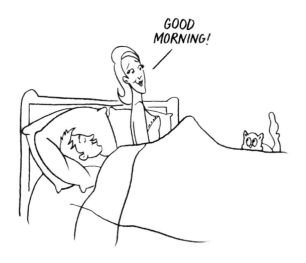

How long till my fella gets up?

If your muscles are a bit out of shape, it can take about 3 months to strengthen them. A Specialist Physiotherapist can reassess your pelvic floor muscle strength at intervals. A sign that your muscles are getting stronger is when you wake up with an erection!

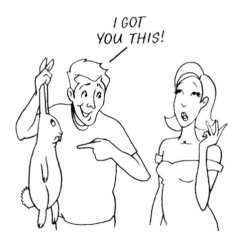

It's good to talk

Your partner might worry that she no longer turns you on.
It can help to talk about it and reassure her that it's a physical
problem and nothing to do with your relationship. Remember
that sex doesn't have to include penetration. You can try all
kinds of other things together like sensual massage or oral sex,
or experimenting with sex toys.

Going to a clinic

Specialist clinics help a great deal. You'll be able to talk to professionals who have experience dealing with erection problems, and they'll be able to assess you and give you advice. It can be helpful to take your partner with you. You can talk to the specialists together and choose the most appropriate treatment method. Whatever you decide to do, keep pumping that pelvic floor! A strong pelvic floor works alongside other treatments and can improve the result you get from them.

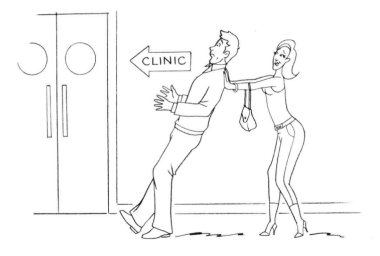

CLINIC

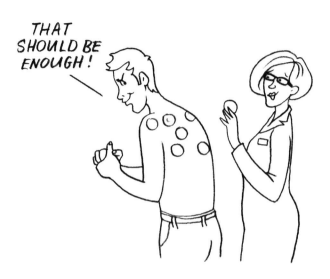

Testosterone patches

If you've a low libido caused by a hormone deficiency, testosterone patches may help you. Your GP may refer you to an endocrinologist who will assess you. Testosterone patches aren't suitable for men with known or suspected prostate or breast cancer.

Sex pill for men

After an assessment your GP or Specialist might prescribe you some pills. Some tablets need to be taken up to an hour before sexual activity. Others can be taken as a daily dose for a more natural response. Oral medication should not be taken with nitrates prescribed for chest pain and can cause side-effects including headache, facial flushing, nasal congestion, and indigestion.

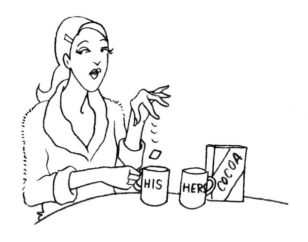

Injections

Another treatment is using an injection to help you get an erection. You will be taught to inject either side of your penis to make it hard. This can have a few side effects, including a burning sensation and prolonged erection. You'll be shown how to do the injections, and your Specialist can talk to you about side effects.

48

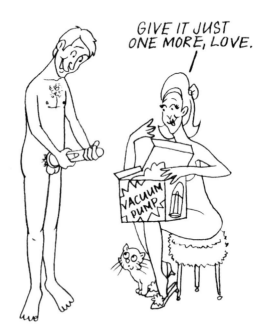

Vacuum therapy

A vacuum pump cylinder is placed over the penis and air is sucked out of the cylinder to form a vacuum. This draws blood into your penis and makes it hard, and there is a constrictive ring to stop the blood escaping. Side effects of this method include feelings of coldness, numbness or pain.

Sexual pain

If sex hurts, don't just put up with the pain. Your GP can assess you for infection and other underlying problems, and offer you treatment. Once that's sorted, a Specialist Physiotherapist can teach you relaxation and use gentle manual techniques that can help.

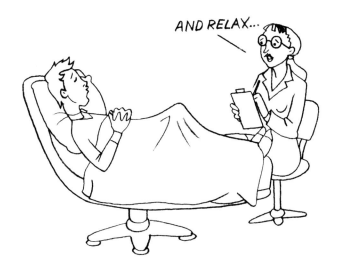

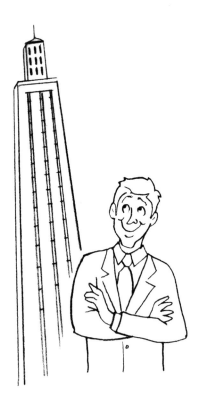

Pump it up!

Every time you exercise your pelvic floor muscles remember that you are making a strong base for your erection. Big buildings need good foundations, so keep pumping!

Where to find a Specialist Physiotherapist

CPPC Chartered Physiotherapists Promoting Continence
c/o The Chartered Society of Physiotherapy
14 Bedford Row
London WC1R 4ED
020 7306 6666
www.cppc.org.uk

**ACPWH Association of Chartered Physiotherapists
in Women's Health**
c/o The Chartered Society of Physiotherapy
14 Bedford Row
London WC1R 4ED
020 7306 6666
www.acpwh.org.uk

Other books by the same author

All books available online at www.yourpelvicfloor.co.uk at £7 + £1 p&p

Stronger and Longer!
Improving erections with pelvic floor exercises

Living and Loving After Prostate Surgery

Use it or Lose it!
Self-help book for men with urinary leakage and erectile dysfunction

Prevent it!
Guide for men and women with leakage from the back passage

Clench it or Drench it!
Self-help book for women with urinary leakage

Make it or Fake it!
Self-help book for women with sexual dysfunction

Love Your Gusset: Making friends with your pelvic floor
A light-hearted little book for women with urinary leakage

Thanks & Links

Expert clinical reviewers:
Kay Crotty MCSP Chartered Physiotherapist
Jennifer Wonnacott MSc BASRT and
UKCP accredited Psychotherapist and
Psychosexual Therapist
Sally Openshaw MSc BASRT accredited
Psychosexual Psychotherapist

Editors:
Martin Dorey
Ana Alteryus
www.copymonkey.biz

Illustrations:
Peter Clover

Design:
Tigerplum
www.tigerplum.com